Duck 'Til Carcinoma

…Navigating the Breast Cancer Experience

by Kathleen Stone, Ph.D.
INSTEAD International

"Do not follow where the path may lead. Go instead where there is no path and leave a trail."

— *Ralph Waldo Emerson*

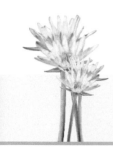
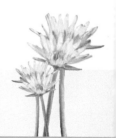

Proceeds from the sale of this book will be donated to organizations involved in the support of breast cancer patients and breast cancer research.

Duck 'Til Carcinoma...
...Navigating the Breast Cancer Experience

Copyright © 2007 Kathleen Stone

Kathleen Stone, Ph.D.
E-Mail: kstoneINSTEAD@aol.com
www.INSTEADinternational.com

First Edition
ISBN: 0-9764279-2-3

An original publication of
INSTEAD International, Burr Ridge, IL, U.S.A.

Printed in the United States of America

Photographs by Kathleen Stone
Design and Layout by Bohringer Creative, Inc. www.bohringer.com

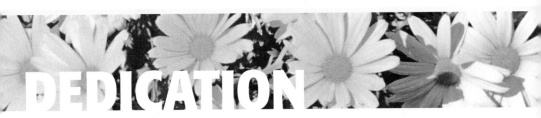

DEDICATION

This book is dedicated to
all the *Courageous Women*
who have been engulfed in
the breast cancer experience,
and to the families,
friends, supporters and
caregivers who have helped
navigate its raging torrent.
To those who have journeyed
beyond our world, you will
never be forgotten. You are
with us always in the Spirit
of Nature & the Universe
that has inspired the poetic
and photographic images
which permeate this book.
To those who are fellow alumna,
We share a unique sisterhood
that makes us all
Powerful Women.

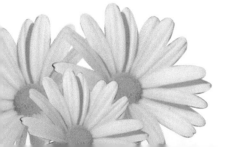

Table of Contents

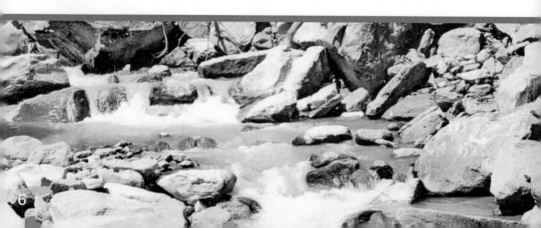

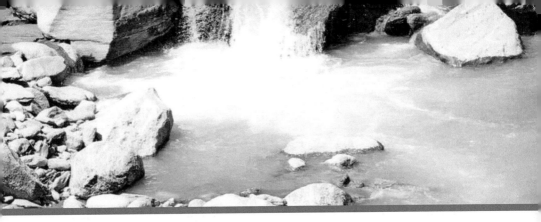

Duck 'Til Carcinoma

There's a little white duck in me
That refused to quack.
She sat back,
And let the mallards prune
Assuming their predominant power.
Until that fateful day,
When carcinoma got in the way!

It's easy to duck from hurt,
Embarrassment, anger, fear.
Safer to hold back, and not quack,
Letting years of emotional carcinomas
Build like insulating feathers,
Like water rolling off a duck's back.
Our down of muffled rage.

Yet carcinoma is a wake-up call,
A summons to alert!
Can't bury my head in the sand.
Can't duck from the painful truth!
A challenge to quack back.
A fight for life.
A time to stretch my neck
And be heard!

INTRODUCTION

Duck 'Til Carcinoma may seem too clever of a title for a book about a serious subject like breast cancer. Please understand that this book is not meant to make light of the breast cancer experience. Breast cancer is truly a journey of a woman's body and soul, and my original poetry shared in this book was written while I was personally feeling all the anguish of this profound transformation. It is my hope that the inspiration shared through my poetry will generate enlightened thoughts and feelings, and help those diagnosed with breast cancer to reflect on the incredible journey of navigating the rocks and rapids that are encountered in this intense process.

I have navigated the various phases of the breast cancer experience as though I have been in a kayak, and I have been launched down a river with swirling, violent rapids. I am hanging on for dear life and "ducking" to avoid being consumed by the intense power of the rapids of carcinoma. I am gripping a paddle, and one side of the paddle is "medical," and the other side is "wholistic." I firmly feel that both are very important in dealing with breast cancer, and I found myself constantly alternating one side of the paddle in the water, and then the other. As I bounce down rushing rapids, the kayak approaches a number of huge boulders. These boulders are the chapters of **Diagnosis, Decisions, Local Control, Adjuvant Therapy,** and the wild ride ending by sailing over a waterfall into the peaceful lagoon of the cancer **Alumni.**

Ductal Carcinoma is the medical term used for breast cancer, and the title of this book takes that term and playfully twists it into the related message of **Duck 'Til Carcinoma**. The poem **Duck 'Til Carcinoma** relates to the shock of life before and after the breast cancer diagnosis. Many of us go along for years, "ducking" from issues to create a sense of comfortable complacency. Suddenly, with the diagnosis of breast cancer, we can "duck" no more, and must face every part of our true Self. Breast cancer forces us to discard part of ourselves, and the past, as we hang on for dear life and ride the kayak of challenges in a profound, transforming present. The poem **Kayak** is designed to show how our life is like different kinds of boats, but the kayak is my best metaphor for life in the breast cancer journey.

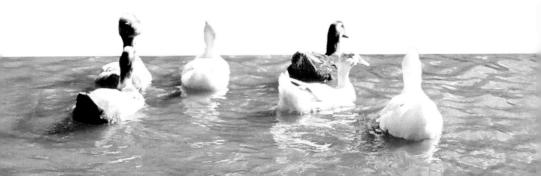

Kayak

Sometimes I'm like a speedboat,
Revving my engine,
With high throttle through a mirror glass lake,
Creating energetic waves that reverberate
Above and below the surface of life.

Sometimes I'm like a rowboat,
Slowly plodding through rippled waters of existence,
In the robotic rhythm of labor.
Aching arms pulling oars of obligation.
Slow progress with restful stops to float.

Sometimes I'm like a canoe,
Gliding lightly along the stream of evolution,
Twisting from right to left,
As the paddle softly rises and dips,
To the smooth accommodation of the moment.

Sometimes I'm like a sailboat,
WIth a sail as effortless power,
Laying back and accepting the wind
As the spiritual source of direction.
An intuitive compass connecting to my course.

Yet when I'm most truly me,
I am like a kayak.
One paddle, one small vessel alone,
Vigorously navigating the rapids of opportunity,
Flowing around every obstacle.
Reveling in the splash of life's joyride!

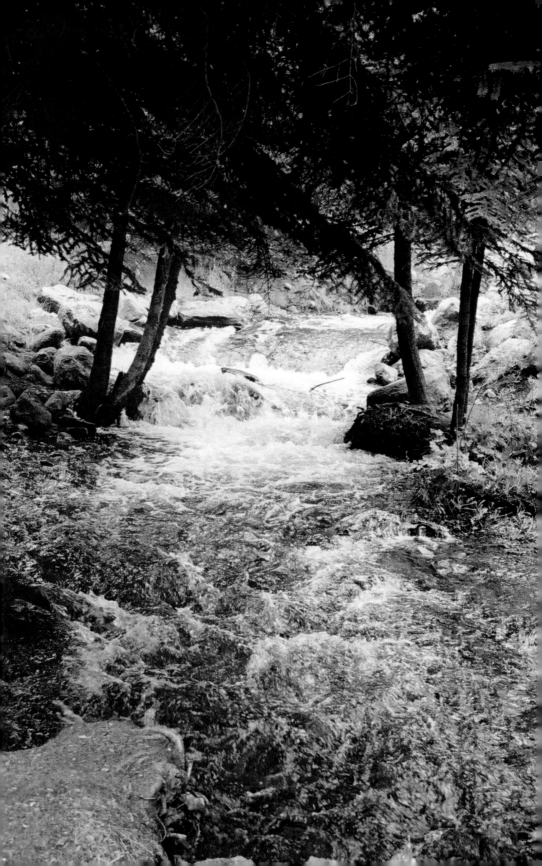

Once You've Found It

Once you've found it,
You've got it!
Doctors copiously use X-rays,
Ultra-Sound, CATS-scans, MRI,
To proactively search for hidden disease
You pray they will not find.

Medical technology spends so much time,
In diligent microscopic examination,
For the illusive maladaptive culprits.
An ominous hope for a clear vision,
No distortion, no collision,
No cautioning provision.

Yet, like a needle in a haystack,
The roulette wheel finally hits....
And you've got it!
Suddenly you're the unlucky one.
Some gamble, risk, unknown reaction,
Has caught up with your health.

And in a single snapshot,
A grim prognosis becomes clear.
Disease is here.
A daunting demon needs dissipating.
Years of relief disintegrating,
Tears of anguish anticipating.

Yes, once you've found it,
You've got it!

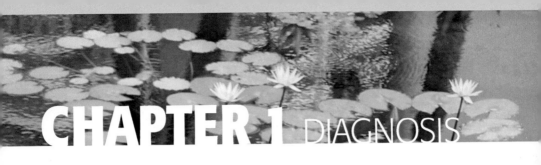

CHAPTER 1 DIAGNOSIS

Once You've Found It

I came across this simple yet profound insight in the early stages of my breast cancer diagnosis: *"Once you've found it, you've got it."* There is so much emphasis related to detecting breast cancer with self-examination and mammograms, that women become intensely fearful about looking for what they are terrified they will find. Having been through that experience, I also felt what it was like to move to the other side of fear, and to be diagnosed with breast cancer.

The technology used for diagnosis was, in itself, a profound experience. Suddenly there were recorded in pictures my breast and its insidious disease. There is an old saying that "a picture is worth a thousand words," and, I can say from experience, that the film evidence of diagnosis leaves one speechless. I have put into intense poetic expression the significant meaning of the **Mammogram** and the **Ultra-Sound.** The mammogram is portrayed as such a daunting experience, that I also wrote a fun, uplifting poem that talks about the upside of the mammogram. It is called **Mammogramma.**

Many of the women who may read this book will fortunately be dealing with an earlier stage cancer that can be resolved with a breast conserving procedure. I was not so lucky. I had the more extensive opportunity to experience all the potential steps in the breast cancer process, included the dreaded mastectomy. The two poems, **Films** and **Radiology Reading** sadly express my experience of loss. I'm certain lumpectomy patients will also identify with their own sense of loss. In a way, my poems are also inspiring, as they show the grief that I felt, and yet they also portray how I was able to move beyond the profound loss. I hope my honesty in these poems helps women to see that there is a life beyond lumpectomy and mastectomy.

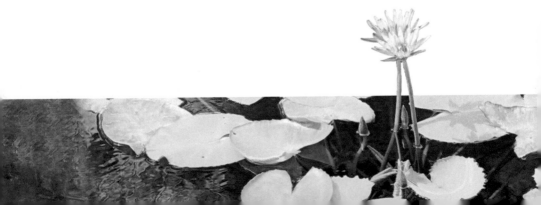

Mammogram

One of a woman's most feared experiences,
A mammogram.
Surrendering one's female body,
The sensual cushion of her heart,
To the daunting micro-examination.

The word "vice" is often used
In sexual innuendo.
Yet the mammo "device"
Is a true mechanical vice,
That entraps a woman's fragile soul.

How humiliating to have one's breast
Clamped within the teeth of the beast,
The soft delicate tissue often left in vulnerable capture
While films are quickly reviewed.
Feeling trapped as a potential victim of insidious disease.

Squish down, "Don't breathe."
Squish sideways, "Don't breathe."
Click picture, click uncertainty.
Screaming inside to be released,
And relieved of the demon for another year!

Medical technology may be life-saving,
But medical examination is soul wrenching.
It's no wonder women approach each year with fear.
For the dreaded uncertain film
Is the deathwatch of the mammogram.

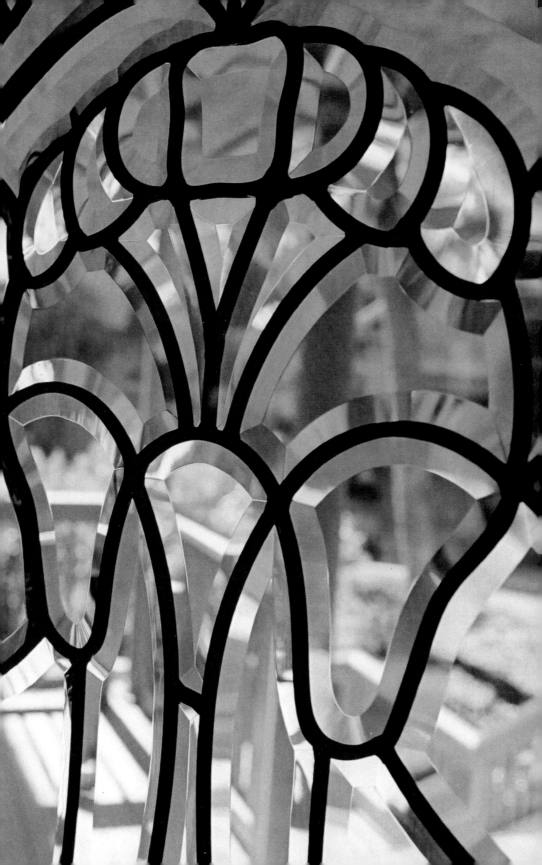

Mammogramma

A honey graham is yummy
When you need a snack to share.
It's fun to get a telegram
From folks traveling here and there.

A funny joyful happygram
Brings a smile to my face.
Especially if there's not a milligram
Of cancer they can trace.

And when I've become a gramma
I'll celebrate with tears,
Each annual clean mammogram,
Relieving recurrence fears!

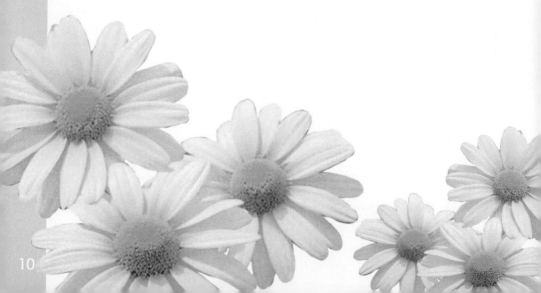

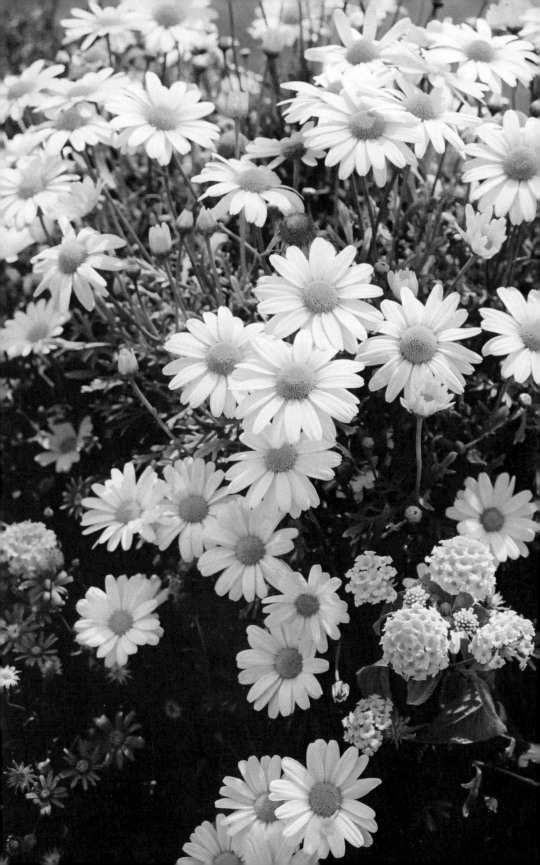

Ultra-Sound

Suddenly my body has become
A microcosm of collaborating cells,
Creating a symphony of health
For an audience of trained technicians.

My physical essence
Has become a molecular marvel,
Being explored across
A finitely revealing T.V. screen!

The sound waves pass through my body,
Exploring the regularity of health,
And marveling at the wonder
Of the female anatomy.

Yet the adventure is foreboding
Within the excitement of a healthy body,
Lies the daunting underlying mission,
Of detecting dis-eased disharmony.

Like the ultimate nightmare of a perfectionist,
Every cell is being examined
In microscopic precision....
Searching for a serious flaw.

How unsettling, how unnerving,
Is the modern diagnosis of physical health!
A supreme screening of inner uncertainty....
The ultra-sound!

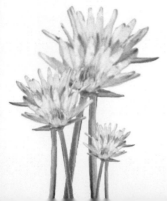

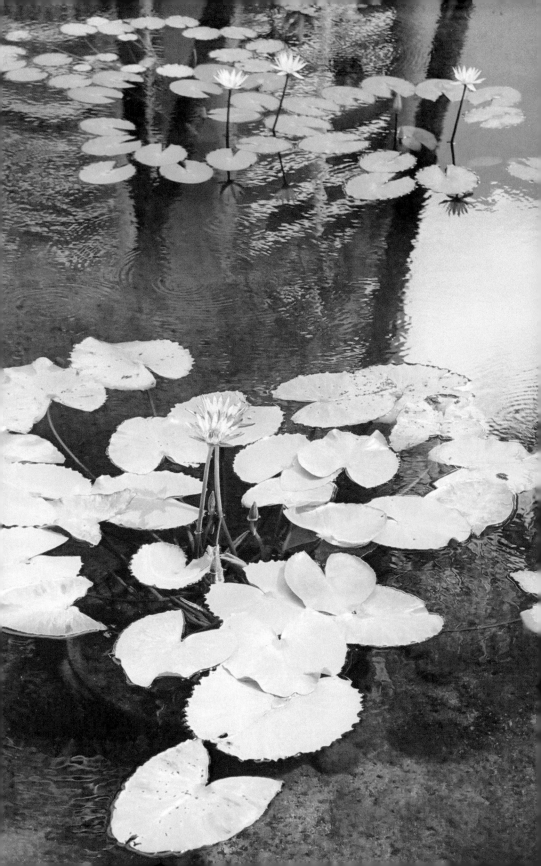

Radiology Reading

A shiny irregular shadow
Ominously glares out,
'Mid a smooth marbleized egg
That once was my left breast.
Comparing the smooth pattern of the right
With the glaring star on the left.
Invasive ductal and lobular carcinoma
Shouts with blatant malignancy.

A magnification view
Shows a grayish web,
And several foreboding spiders,
Arms of the malignant invasion.
Ultrasound confirms a solid mass.
The waves are disturbed,
By a column of darkened distortion,
In the one o'clock position.

Lung x-ray is an additional probe.
No evidence of active lung infiltrate.
No pleural effusion or pneumothorax.
Heart is normal in size.
The day of surgery, a guide wire is inserted,
Marking the center of the targeted carcinoma.

Nostalgia embraces the last radiology images,
Motherly memories of a
Doomed malignant breast.

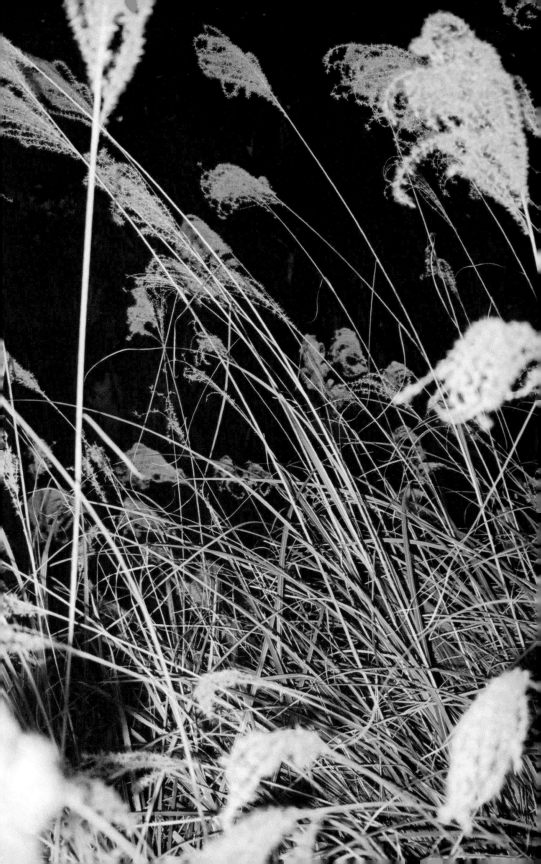

Films

A large brown envelope needs to be returned.
Yet I cannot give it back.
Within are mammogram & ultrasound films,
Used for the surgical decision of mastectomy.

My films....
I look at the first mammogram image,
All that remains of my cherished left breast,
Sacrificed in its death to save my life.

I ponder the white glaring shadow,
The infiltrating star of invasive
Ductal and lobular carcinoma.
Oh, the painful memory of that profound day,
When the surgeon first viewed this evidence
Of dreaded diagnosis.

The marbleized set of ultrasound films,
Again record my breast in its saddened malaise.
The mammogram films from the day of surgery
An invasive guide wire bookmarks my breast
For the awaiting scalpel.

At last, enlightened positive x-rays!
Normal images of lungs, heart and right breast!
Thankfully, no indication of additional tumor,
A prognosis of hope beyond cancer.

Films become priceless records of life's memories,
Weddings, birthdays....surgery.
I hope the hospital archives protect these films.
They are all I have left of an important part of me.

Cancer

Once you are diagnosed with breast cancer, the decisions become overwhelming. First, there is the decision of how you are emotionally going to handle the identity of having cancer. Suddenly people look at you differently. It's hard to have people crying when they see you. You become numb, and still just want to be who you were. The poems *Cancer* and *Label* both put into words the feelings of that profound identity crisis.

Then there are significant decisions related to the local control aspects of biopsy, surgery, and lymph node dissection. These are paralleled with the adjuvant therapy decisions of chemotherapy and radiation. If there is a mastectomy, a woman must suddenly also make an informed decision regarding reconstruction. Then there are decisions related to a second opinion for the various aspects of treatment. All these medical decisions are gut-wrenching as they emotionally and spiritually connect with a woman's soul.

Once I faced the reality of surgery, I found myself feeling like I was being swept off my feet by a whirlwind of decisions. The surgeon did explain that breast cancer is generally slow growing, and that I could take a little time with my decision. Take time! A day, a week…what should I do? I had received the dreadful biopsy results just two weeks before we were to travel overseas on a scheduled vacation to a special Swiss mountain resort in the valley of the famous Matterhorn mountain. I had been visiting the village of Zermatt, Switzerland yearly as my personal spiritual pilgrimage. I agonized over canceling the trip and scheduling the surgery, and listened to my heart for the answer. My heart told me that God was calling me to the mountain first, and that I would find spiritual direction there. I was drained and needed to be strong for the surgery, so I went to the mountain first, to connect with God and gain my strength. The overseas trip delayed the surgery date approximately ten days, and it was one of the best decisions I made in the breast cancer process. This is expressed in the poem *I Went To the Mountain.*

During the time in Zermatt, I hired a Swiss guide who became a living lesson in how God takes care of me. He accompanied me on a treacherous hike, and he kept calmly repeating, *Give Me Your Hand* and *Walk Like An Elephant.* His guidance became my imagery of the entire healing process of the breast cancer journey. I would walk slowly and surely like an elephant, and know that God was guiding every step of my difficult path through the people he sent to help me along the way. The guide was the image of God's hand in caring for me. It set the stage for me to trust each additional hand that supported me through all the decisions regarding my treatment, as well as my emotional healing.

Cancer

Diagnosed with cancer.
The profound reality of fear,
Being given a challenge,
To reach into the depth of soul,
To ignite a fusion of positive energy
That will neutralize the festering beast.

Accepting the label of cancer.
Pleading to the saddened eyes of others…
"Do not pity me!"
But celebrate the wealth of my health,
As it is forced to defend
Against a small army of mutant cells.

Surrendering to the surgery for cancer.
Honoring God's blessing of the surgeon's hands
That guides the gifted scalpel to orchestrate
The dissection of the militant tissue
That invades with destructive disharmony.

Honoring the therapy for cancer.
Chemotherapy is slowly destroying
The unwelcome malignant ones,
While radiation anoints the battlefield scene
With the blessed optimism
Of a lifetime of residual Peace.

Experiencing the shared journey of cancer.
Climbing the jagged path of recovery.
Finding God's hand as my guide,
In the prayers, cards, food, flowers,
And projected positive energy
Of those who cheer each step as I heal.

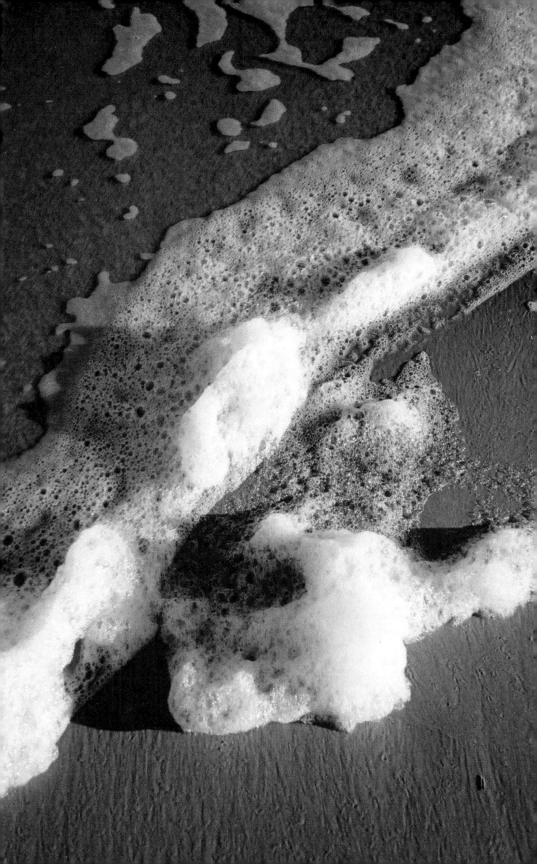

LABEL

Suddenly diagnosed with the dreaded Big "C".
My new identity.
"I'm still me," I cry out!
As sad onlookers pity my new label,
'Mid fading memories of who I really am.

Yes, there was a tumor
That proportionately occupied
Less than 1% of my body.
Yet for 100% of my current life.
The mournful eyes of those around
Now watch me succumb to cancer.

I see it on their stoic faces.
They don't know what to say.
Forcing myself to bravely smile,
I strongly reassure them
That "It's okay, I'm okay, I'll be fine....
It's only cancer."

I hate the label of cancer,
How others perceive me now.
Like I'm contagious, sick, delicate,
With one foot on the road to dying.
Yet over 99% of me is a strong healthy spirit,
Refusing to be overthrown
By the ominous cancer label.

Give Me Your Hand

Give me your hand,

Dear child,

As we walk along a jagged pathway,

Where you might stumble.

Give me your hand,

Fellow traveler,

For the path is narrow,

And the edge is steep.

Give me your hand,

Dear friend,

For there is a dangerous crossing,

And I will guard you with my life.

Give me your hand,

And feel the firm grasp

Of my strong forearm,

That will never let you go.

For I cannot smooth away

The difficult steps of your destiny.

Yet, be assured, that at all times I will be there

To give you my hand and my heart.

I Went To The Mountain

A dire diagnosis,
A foreboding surgical intervention.
Sidetracked along life's progressive journey.
So I went to the mountain.

The mountain majesty has always been
A place to breathe through my soul.
To immerse myself in the essence of God,
Amid the solitude of the most High.

This is not a gentle mountain,
But a powerful granite pyramid,
A physical symbiosis with the Trinity.
Father, Son, and Spirit.

The Father of the mountain
Is in the strength of the rock.
The Son is the human touch of my footsteps.
The Spirit is the song of the brisk, crisp wind.

I climb the jagged pathway,
Inhaling every breath within my core,
Exhaling from the depth of a courageous soul.
Oh, the strain to defy the painful pull of gravity!

I consecrate every cell of my womanly power,
And purge all negative energy.
For the mountain is a magnificent metaphor
Of the strength within me to heal.

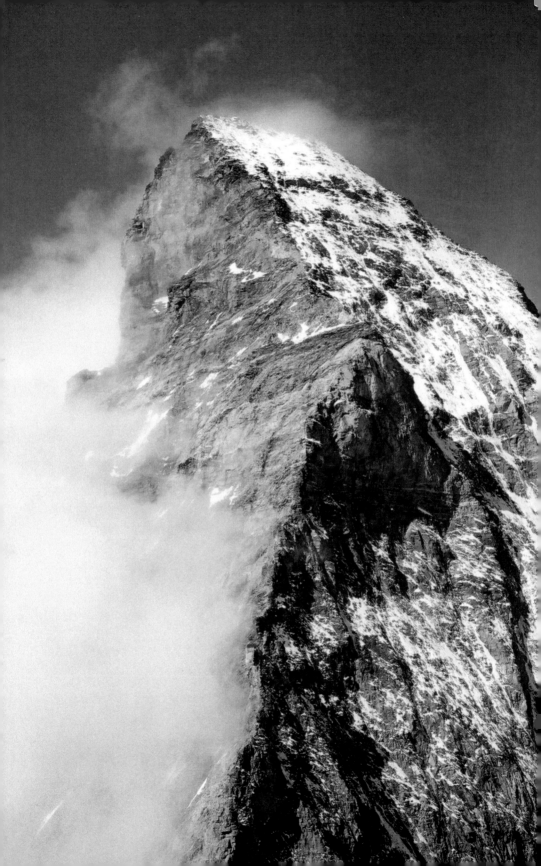

Walk Like An Elephant

Walk like an elephant, my child,

For the journey is long and steep,

And can leave you breathless

In the challenge of this difficult path.

Slowly move one foot forward,

And firmly plant your step

Upon the same safe footprint

That I have left before you.

Heavy, slow step,

Heavy, sure step.

Deep, slow breath,

Deep sure breath.

This is your time of courage.

This is your journey of change.

The past is falling behind you,

As you ascend beyond the horizon.

So put on your heavy shoes of the present,

And your thick skin of protective trust.

Your intuitive trunk is your guide,

As you walk like an elephant.

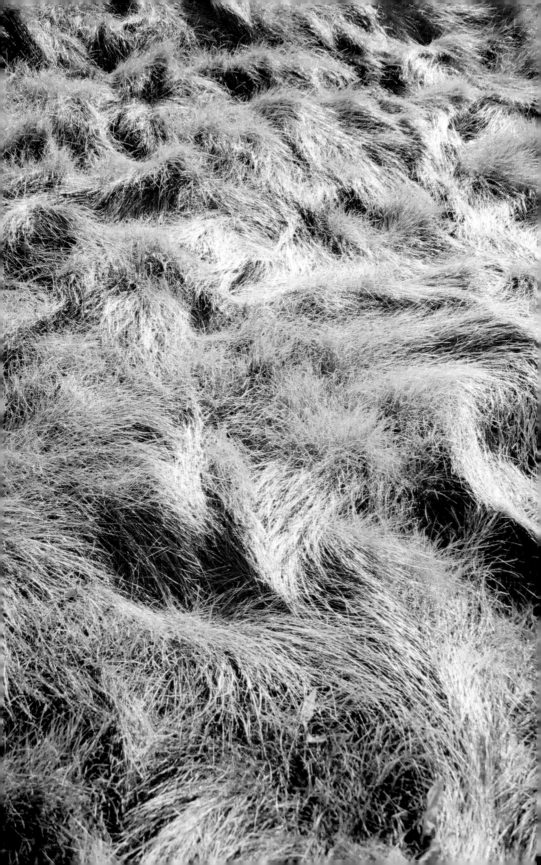

Rising Son…

by James Stone

Three weeks ago I got the call that a son can't ever anticipate,
My mom has been invaded by breast cancer and unknown lies her fate.
At first it seems surreal – like it really isn't true,
But the anguish in my mom's voice made it clear of what she knew.

Since then, in the last three weeks I've focused on the "glass half full,"
But harshly today's reality hit me – my outlook a bunch of bull.
For today I felt the stinging pain and anger of what my mom faces ahead,
The pain of surgery, the radiation and the chemotherapy we all dread.

It's one thing for a person to live a life that leads to bust,
But to happen to a person of integrity and care is unequivocally unjust.
A preacher to us all, a teacher, friend and mentor,
A mom who loves with all she has and one who I adore.

The smartest of us all – a truly gifted, creative mind,
Another who aced her PhD I simply cannot seem to find.
Why do the good suffer, I ask, what purpose can it be,
While criminals from both ghettos and corporate sneak through life scott-free.

As I sat in the room and watched my mom drift in and out of sleep,
Memories raced through my head – the many that I keep.
Times I could make my mom feel better – times I could help and solve,
And then I realized how helpless I am – a challenge to my resolve.

Frustration grew to anger at why she must endure,
A cruel, heartless disease that robs its victims of life so pure.
None of us know what will be the outcome of this stage,
But I will move heaven and earth to help my mom turn the page.

For 30 years my mom has been tied for my biggest fan,
And through her guidance, love and support I've grown into a man.
So today I leave the innocence of yore, knowing clearly what's at stake,
And commit to helping my mom win out – no matter what it may take.

Life without my mom is not an option, angrily screams my voice,
Instead I will help my mom to win, heal, laugh and to rejoice!

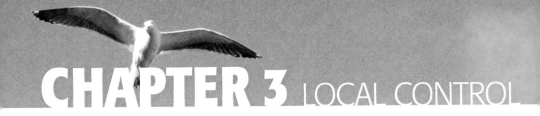

Anesthesia Serenade

Local control is the term that is used to describe the surgical procedures related to removing the breast cancer tumor and lymph nodes. This also includes a procedure called *Sentinel Lymph Node Biopsy*, in which radioactive dye is injected, and there is a mapping of the pathway from the breast to the sentinel lymph nodes. Sentinel lymph nodes can then be removed first, and, if they are negative, there is no need for additional lymph node removal. The sentinel lymph node procedure, mammogram, and insertion of a guide wire for surgery made me truly feel *All Wired Up* by the time I was wheeled into the operating room for my lumpectomy surgery.

In order to create an appropriate supportive atmosphere for myself in surgery, I had requested that music be played, and I had selected the lovely music from the soundtrack of the movie *Rudy.* I had read that a person still can hear during anesthesia, and I wanted my spirit to be uplifted during the surgical procedure. I describe that very positive empowering experience in the poem *Anesthesia Serenade.* My surgeon was wonderful, and fully cooperated and seemed to understand the positive meaning of my request. My surgeon listened with compassion to the anguish with which I approached and surrendered to both surgeries and, like the Swiss mountain guide, he walked like an elephant in the way he guided me to slowly but surely proceed with the necessary and painful surgery decisions. I wrote the poem *Hero* to recall how my surgeon had become another hand of God, like the mountain guide, who had coached me to "Walk like an elephant" to climb the challenging mountain path.

The mastectomy surgery was extremely difficult for me to accept, and it was through a synchronistic recommendation that I was connected with Deena Metzger's book and poster called *Tree.* Deena's powerful image of a woman with a mastectomy scar covered with a tattoo of a tree branch became the most significant way for me to visually look at my second surgery as a powerful experience of my own female transformation. This mastectomy experience is expressed through the poem *Tree.*

During the long waiting time of the first surgery, my adult son wrote a poem that expressed his anguish at seeing his mom go through breast cancer surgery. His feelings are profoundly expressed in the poem *Rising Son*…

Sentinel Lymph Node Biopsy

Sentinel lymph nodes,
Guardians watching and protecting the gatepost.
The aggressive centurions of disease
Yearn to break the barrier
And spiral malignant havoc.

The command post of nuclear medicine,
A tenuous slab on a gurney.
Rolled under the technological tube,
Waiting to be microscopically viewed,
Mapping the enemy's invasive path.

Four wasp-like stings inject radioactive dye
Into the trusting breast.
The body a living monitor,
Tracing the mammary highway
To the critical sentinel outposts.

To lay in watchful silence,
While emitting gamma rays
Into a scintillation detector.
Recording the radioactive journey,
Targeting sentinels for the impending scalpel.

My body has been a willing field,
Fueled by an uncertain optimism.
Has cancer reached the gateposts?
I champion the naïve trust
That negative sentinel signals
Will lead to a positive outcome.

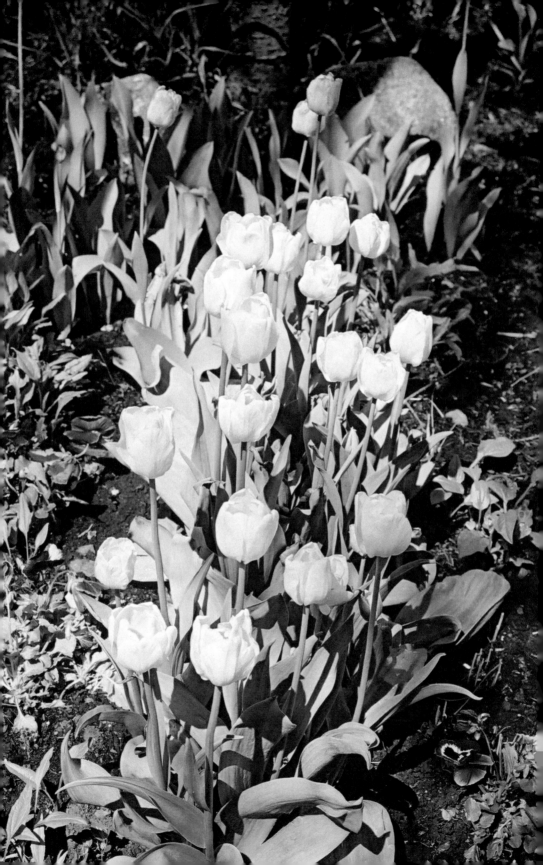

All Wired Up

Surgical preparation
Guided by technology.
A probe wire enters the breast,
And marks the playing field,
That will connect mammogram images
To the searching scalpel.

Nuclear Medicine,
Injecting radioactive dye,
Following the mammary map
To the sentinel lymph node signals.
A geiger beeping pathway
Loudly reverberates at the surgical target.

Wheeled on a gurney shuttle
From mammo moments,
To X-ray explorations.
From nuclear networking,
To the swinging doors of the surgical arena.
All wired up.

All wired up!
They have often said that of me…
That I'm all wired up!
I've always been a "live wire."
Now I'm living proof!
All wired up is my surgical truth!

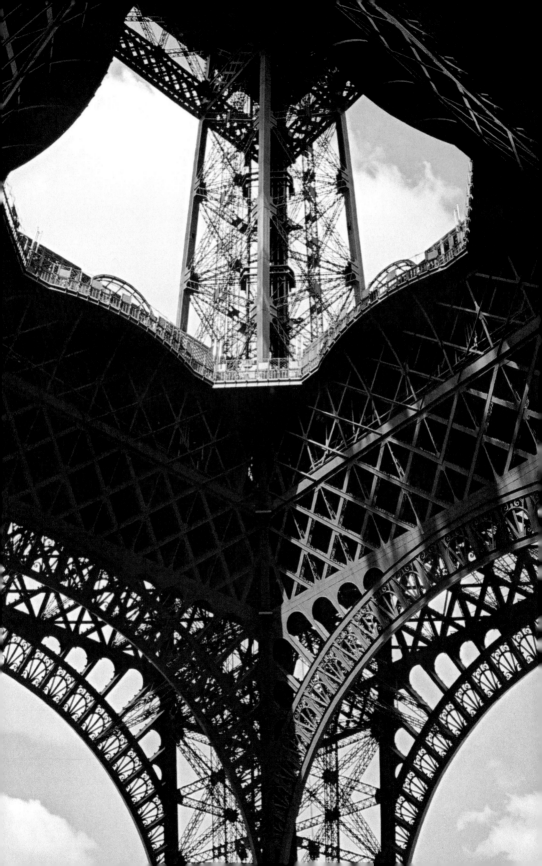

Anesthesia Serenade

Being put to sleep.
An unsettling projection
Of being totally out of control,
While the surgeon cuts into
The precious padding over my heart.

They say one can hear during anesthesia,
Although listening is in the subconscious.
So I select a significant serenade
That will enchant the surgical sanctuary,
And soothe the strings of my trusting soul.

"Rudy, Rudy, Rudy…"
The lilting movie soundtrack
Of an inspiring story
That is the essence of my spirit.
Overcoming adversity, tenacity, not giving up,
Believing passionately in an impossible dream.

In subconscious submission,
My body guides the scalpel of healing incision.
The Rudy serenade integrates the melodic waves
Of soft strings, tenuous horns, Irish rhythms,
And the climactic crescendo of the kettle drum.

A tube is intruding the windpipe of my song,
While machines bear the labor of my breath.
I am numb from pain, yet fully alive in the process.
For I am not a helpless surgical victim.
But a spiritual dancer in flow
With the orchestration of anesthesia.

Tree

"You've got to read Deena Metzger,"

Intuited the wise woman doctor.

She understood well the anguish.

The impending mastectomy

Had imploded within my womanly soul.

This unwelcome spiritual transformation.

Had led me to discover "Tree."

Deena Metzger's book, "Tree" shares her pain,

Her struggle with rage and sensual sacrifice.

Surrendering a breast for her life,

The strength of the Universe

Emerged in her power.

The design of a tattoo on her mastectomy scar

A branch, green leaves, grapes, and a bird.

Her "Tree," forever connecting

Her arm with her heart.

Now is the time for my personal tree,

As I tenderly honor my surgical scar,

A lanced tribute to the feminine spirit.

Defying the constraint of a prosthetic stereotype

I envision a symbolic tattoo...

An olive branch with a pure white dove.

The outward symbol

of Peace within my soul.

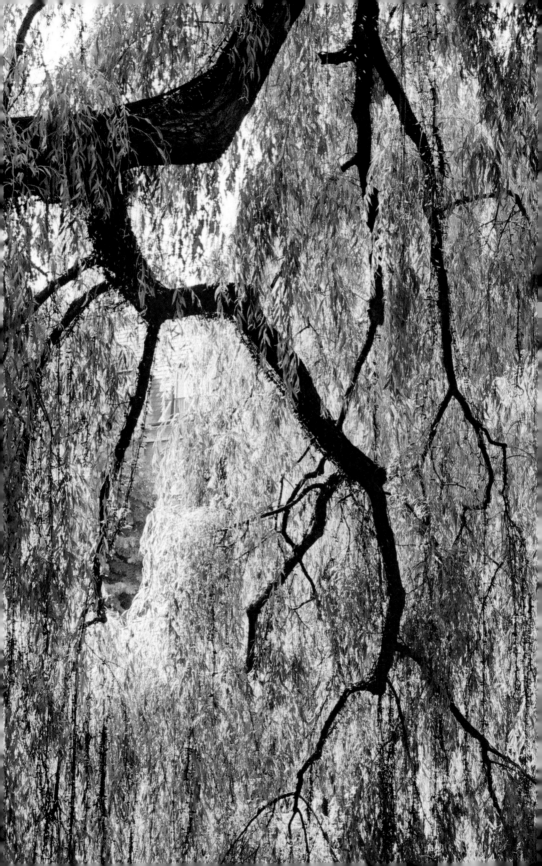

HERO

Has climbed medical mountains
The hero I know so well.
Hundreds of times, he's conquered
In guiding his sacred scalpel.

Patiently listening to uncertainty,
Balancing care and caring.
Guiding the frightened patient
To trust the truth he is bearing.

He consults with calm compassion,
Speaks with a rhythmic song.
Walks cautiously like an elephant,
In the delicate surgical marathon.

He has the soul to inspire,
Never shares arrogance.
Strength and stability in a boyish smile,
Integrity and truth in his stance.

With the gift of youthful experience,
The humility of wisdom beyond his years,
He heals with the heart of a hero.
As he comforts my soul and my tears.

My Hero,
My Surgeon!

Melted Ice

Adjuvant therapy refers to the therapeutic cancer treatments of chemotherapy and radiation. I again had the opportunity to experience both of these treatments. Throughout the course of the breast cancer experience, I was determined to stay very positive, and I did everything I could to integrate positive thinking and visualization to eradicate the cancer from my body. One of the most helpful visualizations I created for myself was the image of *Melted Ice* as a way to see the cancer tumor and cells evaporating into thin air. I also used the experience of playing racquetball by myself, and night after night hitting the ball against the wall as a visualization of destroying cancer cells. That proactive strategy is expressed in the poem *Having A Ball.*

I had a very difficult time surrendering to the process of chemotherapy. I was especially frightened to learn that one of the chemo drugs prescribed for me can have the side effect of damage to the heart. I was relieved to have the *MUGA* test available to assure me that my heart would be protected. The poem *Chemotherapy* was written the morning right before I went in for my first chemo treatment, and it poignantly shows the *anguish* I was feeling at surrendering to this dreaded process. After having become accustomed to the chemo process, I wrote the poem *Chemo* as a way to keep my sense of humor, while fully integrating the profound meaning of this very serious experience.

The chemotherapy regimen prescribed for me was Adriamycin and Cytoxin, or AC, which practically guarantees loss of hair. The hair loss was the worst part of the breast cancer experience for me. I had always had long brown hair, and now I was not only losing my treasured hair, but I felt like my identity was being ripped away from me. The loss of hair was expected to begin on day 14 after the first chemo treatment, and on days 11 through 13, I literally anguished and wrote the most sorrowful poetry to deal with the grief and humiliation at the loss of my hair. The poem *A Head of the Game* deals with my decision to accept the chemo treatment even though I knew it would lead to the hair loss. *Long Tresses* talks about what my long hair has meant to me all my life. The poem *Armageddon* portrays the depth of devastation I felt at the prospect of losing my beloved long hair and accepting the reality of impending baldness.

In the process of radiation therapy, I again had to surrender my total being to the reality of my body being bombarded with dreaded radiation. The poem *Radiant Beauty* shares my acceptance of the process. I had read that the lead chamber for radiation therapy was quite ominous, but the *Lead Vault* in my hospital was actually a rather pleasant cloister. Lying on the table day after day made me feel like I was a *Grocery Sack.*

Armageddon

To each an Armageddon,
A challenge in life
That puts us face to face
With our own personal symbol
Of a fear as strong as death.

For me it was cancer,
And so I was diagnosed with ductal carcinoma.
For me it was a mastectomy,
And twice I faced the scalpel,
Surrendering to a woman's greatest fear.

Now I approach the seemingly final conflict.
Succumbing to the need for chemo,
I entered the toxic battlefield,
Knowing the residual of the medical napalm
Will strip me of my cranial pride.

My next Armageddon is at hand.
Within days, hours, impending baldness.
The emperor has no clothes.
The princess has no hair.
Voices of laughter ring in my ears.

I will look so strange to the world.
Not like the rest…a freak.
My soul hears echoes of ridicule,
As I come to understand my worst Armageddon,
The power of judgment on myself.

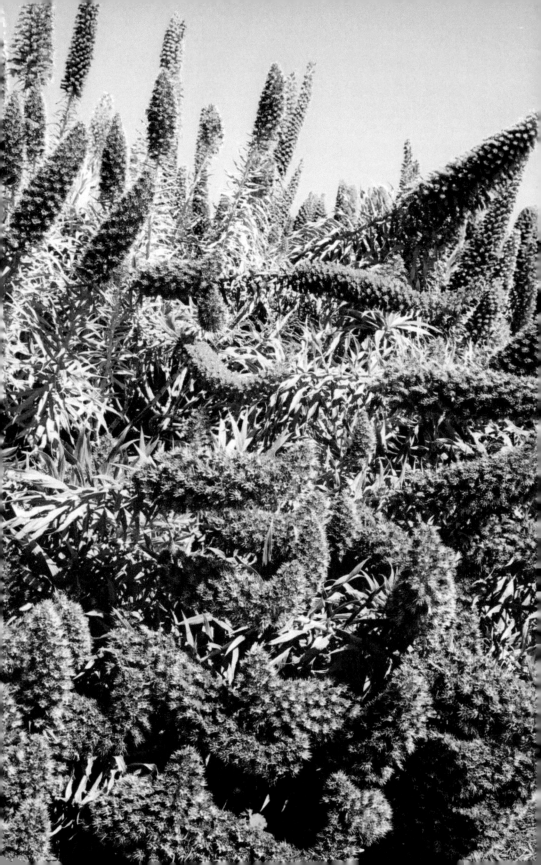

Melted Ice

Tumor and its fragmented messengers
Have attacked my vulnerable breast.
Like the D-Day invasion,
I am responding with all the forces of my soul.

My body engages my threatened immune system
To destroy the malignant masses.
My mind and spirit spring into action,
With the power of visualization.

The cancerous onslaught like a sudden ice storm.
The tumor like an ice cube,
The fragments like malignant chips,
Infiltrating the vessel of my essence.

My mind becomes the most powerful sunlight,
Heating, destroying the unwelcome intruders.
Like an ice cube set on the pavement,
I imagine it melting with the absorption
Of brilliant solar rays.

For what I truly see in my cancer cure.
Is a vision of its slow, total disintegration…
Like ice melting, pooling and evaporating,
Vaporizing, every so gradually, into nothing.

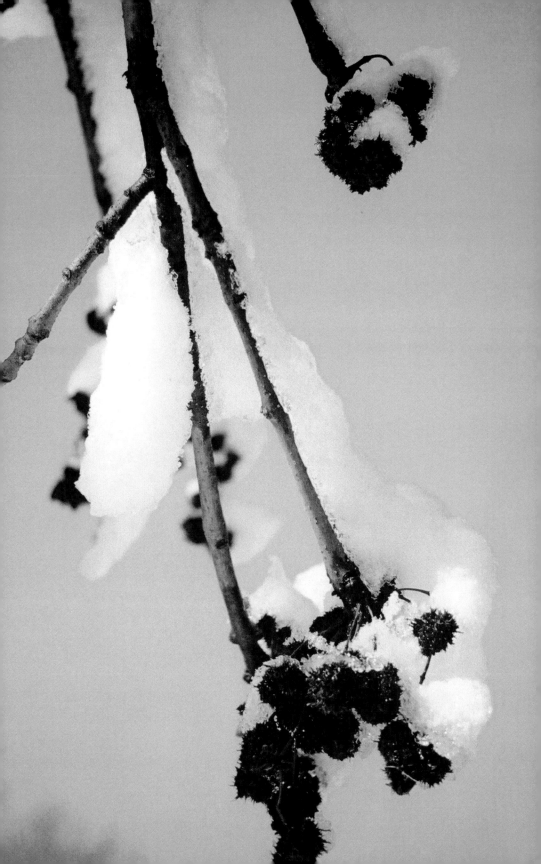

M.U.G.A.

I cried out to the oncologist,
"The fear of Adriamycin
Killing the disease of my breast,
Must not damage my heart."
And he said....."MUGA."

I painstakingly reviewed volumes of research,
And worried about each side effect,
Wondering how treating the bad
Could lead to worse.
And my oncologist reassured me....."MUGA."

I am so worried about myself!
What will become of me?
So much uncertainty!
My heart grieving and breaking,
As I went to the hospital for.....MUGA.

MUGA.....
Multi-Uniform-Gated Acquisition.
Nuclear Medicine watching my aching heart.
Thousands of pictures frame a cardiac cinema.
Medical protection with gamma ray scrutiny.

The heart-wrenching fears of cancer.
The heartfelt medical caring.
Building trust in my heart and soul,
That I will be protected
With the peace of mind of....MUGA!

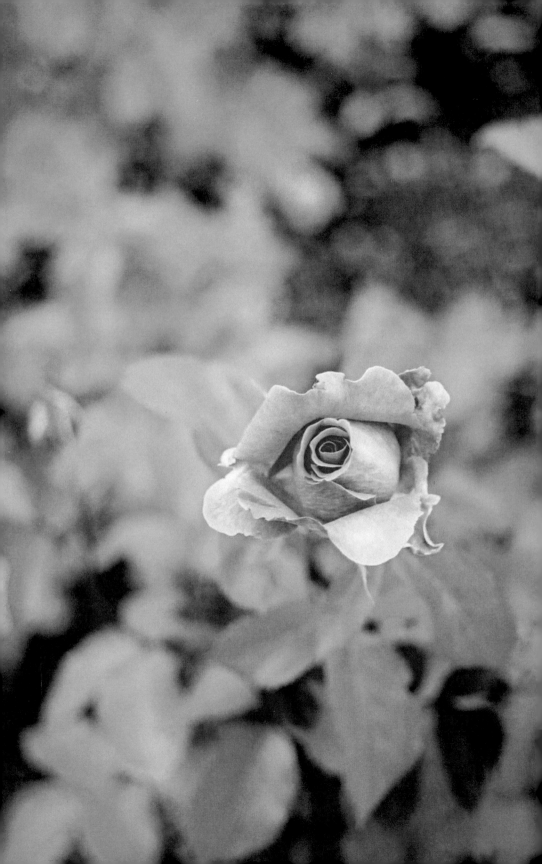

Chemotherapy

My first chemotherapy…
I am engulfed by a death experience.
Ominous oncology.
Injecting medical napalm into my veins
To destroy a covert guerrilla army
Of fragmented sniper cancer cells.

Death to the malignant ones,
Yet death to my innocent healthy cells,
That I have for so long protected and honored.
Now I must surrender my vulnerable body,
To the horror of chemical warfare,
And risk suffering and emotional agony
For the prognosis of a new tomorrow.

Losing, losing, loss.
My good cells are sacrificed.
My vitality at risk,
To withstand the therapy of chemo onslaught.

I touch the silky strands of my hair,
Caressing the long-beloved crown on my head,
Ceremoniously soothing my cranial identity
That is now programmed for a tearful good-bye.

I am dying from within….
My cells, my life force, my hair,
Victims to an insidious force that arose through my cells,
And now will hopefully be destroyed through the ravages
Of……
Chemotherapy.

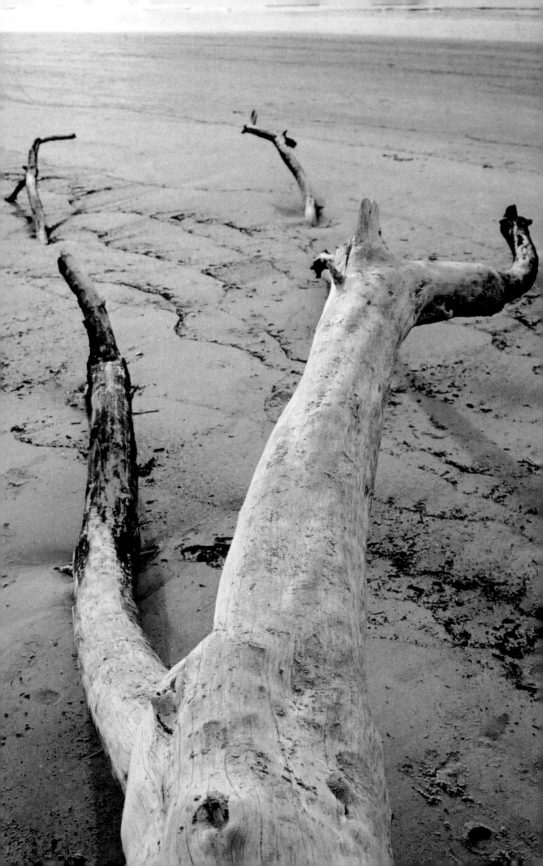

Chemo

I despise the term "Chemo."
It reminds me of a mispronounced acronym
For a Las Vegas game of chance.
Yet perhaps that is truer than we wish to admit.
For chemotherapy is a big gamble for life…
A bet that a highly toxic napalm
Can destroy all sniper cancer cells
Covertly trying to spread insurrection
Within the innocent community of my body.

I hate the risk factor jargon of chemo,
Betting on odds as to cancer's recurrence,
And hedging the bet with the potency of toxin.
The five year survival rate figures
Make my life sound like an uncertain financial investment,
Or, better yet, a new car warranty.
Yet, they give new cars a more assured lifetime
Than the prognosis language of cancer.
No wonder the fear and depression!

Chemo is a trite nickname for a truly lifelong decision.
It relates to the hope for a future,
And the destruction of insidious wild cancer cells.
There are killer cocktails over extended time,
Or blasting with quick heavy hitter bombardment.
The side effects are notorious and often humiliating.
The alternative risks are debilitating.
A gamble with one of the highest stakes in life….
Chemo

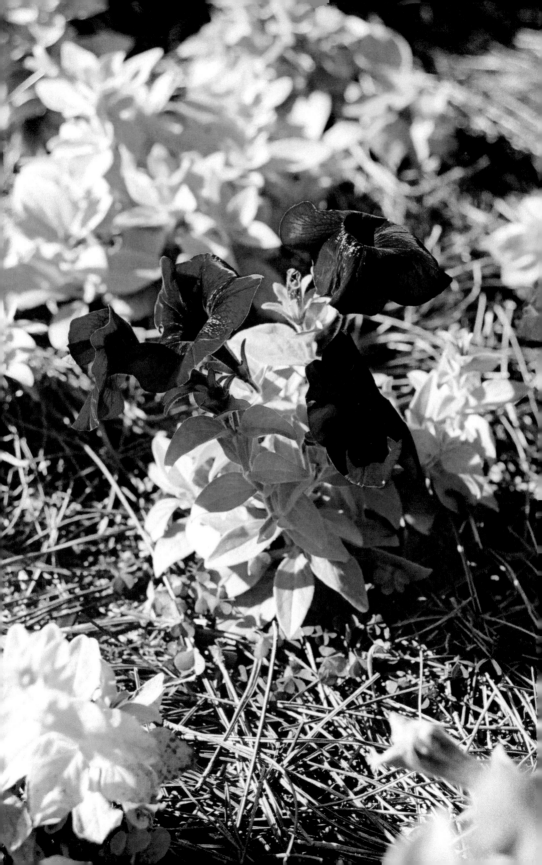

A Head of the Game

The game of beating cancer.
Best odds with strongest toxins,
That also destroy the hair.
A gamble of enduring short term humiliation,
For best odds of long term cure.

Heads or Tails?
Tails….I may tail behind in odds.
Heads…I go ahead with the best,
And know getting ahead at the game,
Means losing a head of hair.

So it's day one treatment.
Toxin rushing into cells,
Shunting the production of protein.
Hair shaft weakened under the skin.
Ready to break upon emerging.

They say it takes from 14 to 17 days.
A somber time of waiting.
Washing, brushing, combing for the last time.
Trying to imagine the unimaginable.
Bawling at the prospect of balding.

Soon day 14 approaches.
Holding scissors, putting them down.
To control the inevitable,
Or wait for nature's ax to fall.
The risk of the game.

It's fine to be ahead of the game,
To arrogantly stay in control.
Yet there's something to be said
For God's timing in the next cancer play.
And honoring my heart….as well as my head.

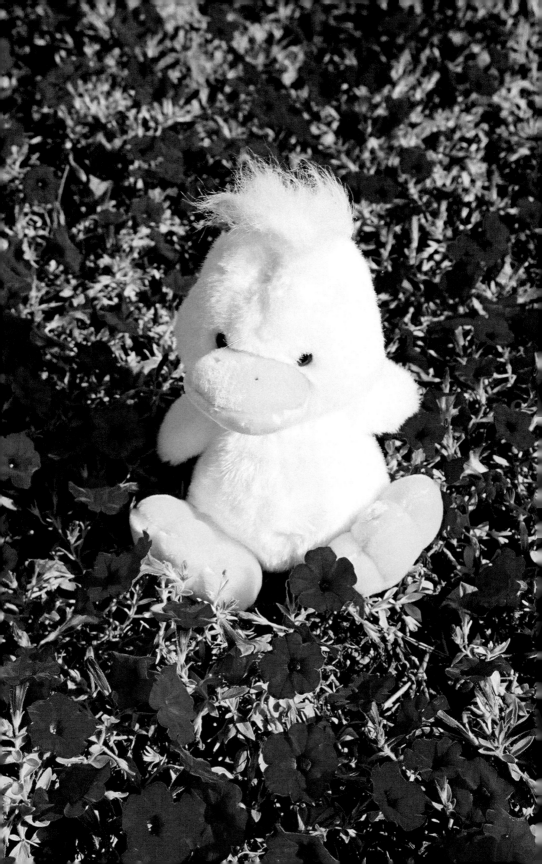

Long Tresses

The beauty of long tresses
A symbol
Motherhood and chocolate pie
Grown years ago
And lovingly maintained over time.
Shafts have broken.
Ends have split.
Yet I have refused trims
And trendy hairstyles
To savor my cherished crown
Of silky tresses,
My personal girlish treasure.
There is something about long hair
That is sensual, womanly,
Flowing, ever growing,
Rebelliousness against stiff conformity.
It's my need to fly with the wind.
My natural identity
That is not rigid,
That enjoys a chameleon touch.
Perhaps it's the sense of free spirit
That is the key,
Or is it the actress and model
That has a passion for beauty?
I have lived with years of princess magic.
Rapunzel, Maid Marion, Angel, Cher…
Nurturing my feminine archetype.
And now my hair loss is eminent.
Yet its phantom essence can never leave my soul.
For I trust the memory of my silky halo
Will sustain my tenacious spirit
In the temporary baldness of chemotherapy.

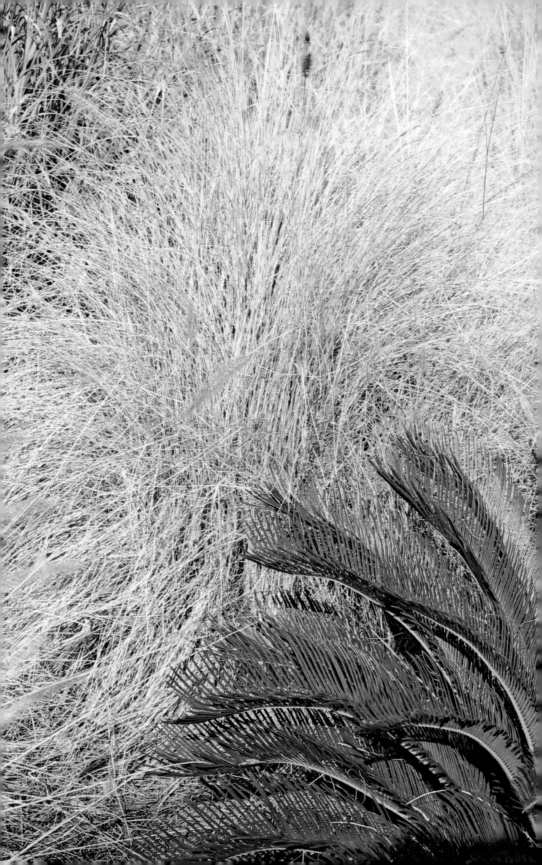

Having A Ball

I had a ball in my hand,
In the hospital after breast surgery.
And I squeezed and squeezed,
Feeling a sense that I still had some control.
Hadn't lost my tenacious childlike spirit,
In a time when I felt I had sacrificed
An important part of my womanhood.

I had a ball in my hand,
As I looked at the orange vial of chemo toxin.
Then I put on my headphones with rock music,
And squeezed and bounced the ball,
To the rhythm of the beat,
As the toxin was pushed into my vein,
Attacking my hair follicles in its cellular invasion.

I have a ball in my hand
Each night, as I fight!
Neither nausea nor fatigue
Keep me away from the racquetball court,
Where I pound the ball against the wall,
Visualizing destroyed cancer cells
With each powerful onslaught.

I have a ball in my hand,
As I don my compression sleeve
On an airline flight out of sight.
No, Cancer has not stopped me!
I live the spirit of the athlete!
In the fright and fight of a lifetime,
You might even think.....I'm having a ball!

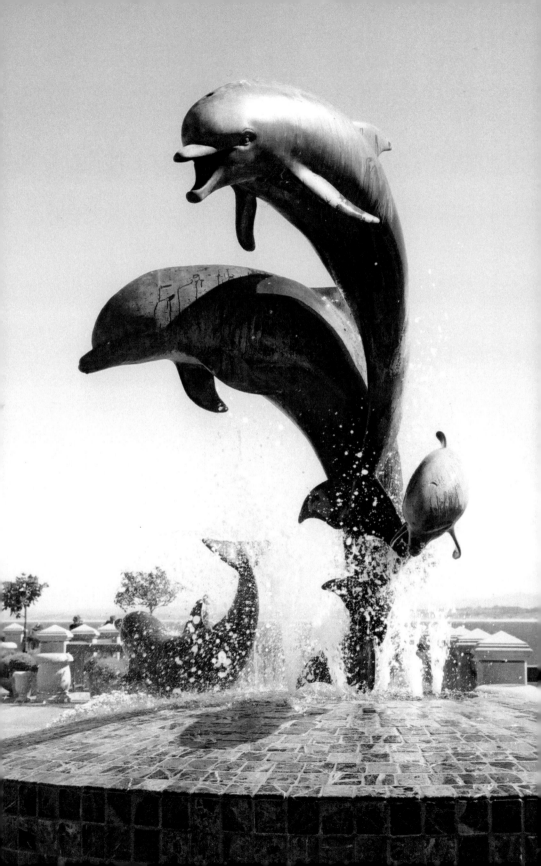

Radiant Beauty

Like a baby,
I now have an alpha cradle
That was poured and hardened
To welcome my unique contour.

As I slide into my prescribed form,
I recline like a mannequin,
Seductively raising my arm,
Awaiting the caress of healing radiation.

Some days require a diaper drape,
A bolus designed to spread
An even, shallow penetration
Of the powerful formulated rays.

Tattoos define my body's target field,
As directed crimson lasers
Beam the coordinates of alignment
For the multi-leaf collinator blocking my vulnerable heart.

The gantry looks like a huge space-age kitchen appliance
That hums when its penetrating rays
Strike at two o'clock,
Then rotate to my eight o'clock body position.

Arcs radiate from front and behind.
My reddened and tanned chest
Is glowing with radiant beauty
In the bombardment of cancer's residual glitter.

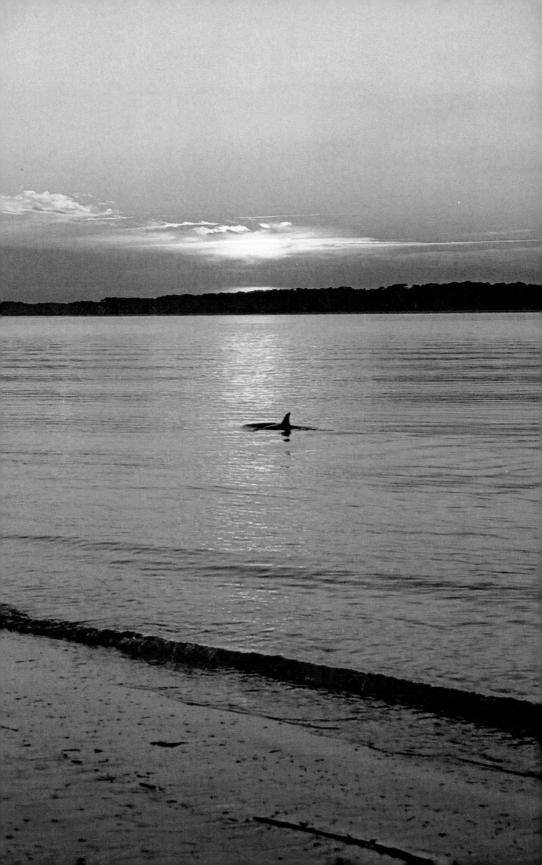

Grocery Sack

Here I am...

Feeling like a large stuffed grocery sack,

Lying on a stalled conveyor belt,

As I contemplate the stillness

Of the next radiation treatment.

A beam of scarlet laser light

Registers my identity.

The tattoos on my chest a bar code

Being carefully scanned for my alignment.

It's an immobile experience,

This radiation business.

My body is a waiting lump,

Like a bump, on a log,

Or a sunning frog.

Yet the stillness of my contour

Disguises the rapture of my silent spirit.

For within this grocery sack of my physical body

Radiates silent celebrating cells

Waving adieu to my vanishing carcinoma.

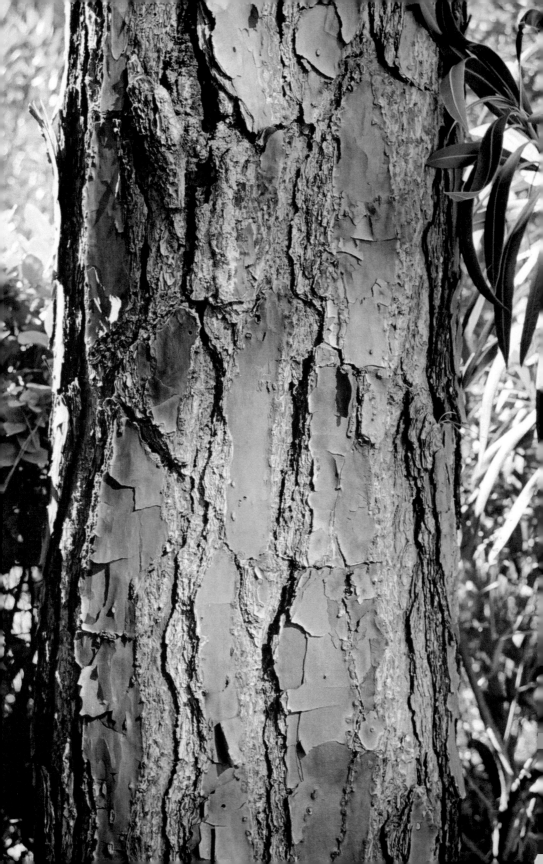

Lead Vault

Hah! Those frightening cancer books
Describe the ominous chamber of radiation.
Beware of the solitary slab
Where technicians scurry to hide behind leaded walls.

But is it lead,
Or do I take the lead?
Is it a vault,
Or do I vault beyond?

The radiation chamber entrance is a marbleized rampway,
Deceptively welcoming with Grecian Ionic pillars.
I am majestically welcomed into the healing arena
Clothed in a turquoise drape.

The lead palace has a mural at my feet,
A tropical waterfall of healing tranquility.
White cubicles line the periphery,
Hiding the current inventory of human alpha cradle forms.

The floor shines in horizontal hardwood veneer.
The whitened walls welcome my spirit.
I am in the lead within the lead chamber,
As I radiantly vault beyond....
With the healing treatment for cancer.

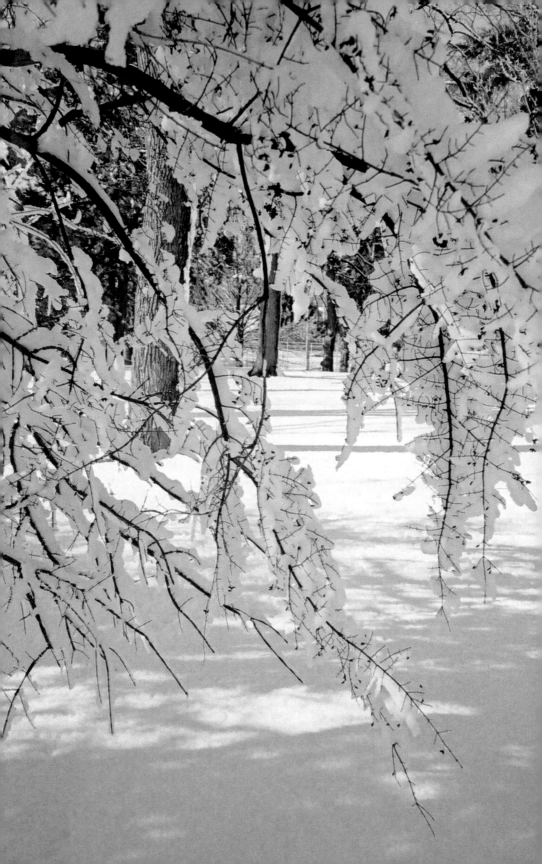

Fine Line

How amazing that the beam of radiation

Targets my chest wall,

Yet misses my heart!

The master of radiation archery,

My radiation oncologist,

Taught me the lesson

Of the fine line.

Cancer has been the supreme journey

of the fine line.

From achieving surgical margins,

To the marginal warning

Of a low white blood cell count.

From the chest tattoo target,

To the arc of demarcation

For a fine radiation beam.

Surviving cancer is the gift of the fine line,

Walking a thin high wire,

Grateful for medical precision,

And trusting the medical team

Weaving its technological wisdom

When life seems to be

Hanging by a thread.

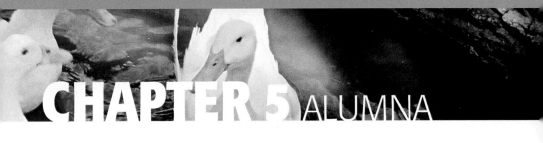

Powerful Woman

It was rather ironic that I had been at a point in my life where I was struggling with my higher purpose. I had completed my doctorate in the spring of 2000, and had become committed to cross-cultural understanding through the completion of an extensive international dissertation research project that had connected me with over 20 universities in ten countries. My dissertation was dedicated to **World Peace and Cross-Cultural Understanding.**

With the profound tragedy of September 11th, 2001, I was stunned and paralyzed as to what one person could do to contribute to peace in this increasingly hostile world. At the time of September 11th, I wrote the poem **Powerful Woman** and sent it out on the INTERNET as my personal plea for world peace. I also attended at that time a workshop called "Journey of Spiritual Transformation." The activities from the day involved soul-searching and the formation of my personal mission statement: **To reflect on the world, discover clever alternatives, and work with visionaries to create Peace.** How ironic that exactly nine months after the creation of my mission statement, my goal emerged from a pregnant incubation, and was born through my diagnosis of breast cancer! It seems profound to think that this cancer experience and writing this book are part of my path leading to fulfillment of my mission statement. It seems as though cancer may have transformed me into one of the powerful women that I tenaciously called forth at the time of September 11th to help the world find a way to peace through feminine power.

I have chosen to call myself a cancer **alumna** (female singular of alumni) rather than use the term cancer **survivor.** The term survivor seems too passive for me, and throughout the breast cancer process, I have been learning, working, battling cancer, with a level of tenacity that has made the memory of my doctoral dissertation seem easy in comparison. I may have had breast cancer, but breast cancer never had me. There is nothing I have done in my life that comes near to drawing on the courage I have used to deal with breast cancer. The poem **Anguish** provides some level of

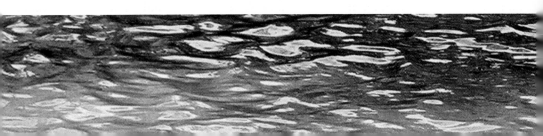

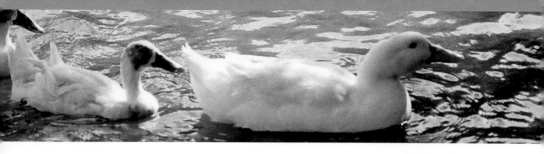

insight into the emotional struggle. *Hair Extension* addresses the profound challenge to my identity. *Trans Am* and *Rear View Mirror* are parallel poems that provide insight into how I used the metaphor of my powerful sports car as my emotional therapy in connecting with my own personal power to beat breast cancer. The poem *Sampson* shares how I have cleverly adjusted to my mastectomy, and was still able to maintain my sense of humor.

Once cancer was behind me, and I had celebrated the one-year anniversary of my diagnosis, I began to reflect more deeply on the profound experience of breast cancer. It had involved seven long months of wearing a wig, before I finally had enough hair to appear in public with my very short haircut. My hair had grown back with lovely varied shades of dark brown, and the hair had *Curls.* I began saying to everyone that "God is my hairdresser." The poem *Fog* was written as a direct experience of driving in a thick fog one early spring morning off the coast of South Carolina. The terrifying experience of driving with my hands tightly gripping the steering wheel crystallized what my life had been like through the year of cancer. Likewise, the direct experience of *Waiting* over an hour before takeoff on a airline flight made me aware of how cancer puts one's life in a holding pattern. The poem *Backwards* was written as I was traveling on a train and reflecting back over a most profound year.

I celebrated the one-year anniversary of my diagnosis by returning to Zermatt, Switzerland, where I felt God's inspiration delivered to me as I watched the sun set on the Matterhorn. The poems *You Came to Me* and *I Understand* express that spiritual inspiration. The poem *I Have Been Healed* was actually written in Zermatt before my first surgery, and it expressed the faith in healing that I had from the time of diagnosis, and that healing has now been transformed into the message that I share personally with my breast cancer *alumni!* Finally *"How Sweet It Is"* reflects the endearing gratitude and admiration toward my medical oncologist.

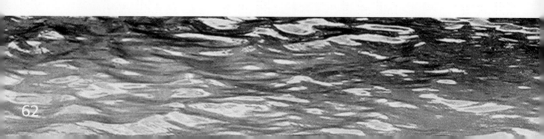

Powerful Woman

Somewhere out there
Is a woman of power…
Biding her time,
While male world leaders
Control the chessmen,
And steadily exert their manly aggression
In worldly power struggles
Over land, oil, wealth….and dogma.

The woman of power
Synergizes the energy
Of powerless women and children.
The lone queen
Will not become a pawn.
She will speak with one voice,
For the hearts of many.
She is the soul of the eternal mother,
The soul that has mourned
The loss of husbands, brothers, sons,
Across the battlefields of time.

The woman of power
Will unite women and shepherd children,
In one worldwide symphony.
A chorus of PEACE!
An echo 'round the world.
Harmony will overcome discord.
She knows the time to speak,
To haunt male aggression
With the tears of history.
The woman of power
Speaks for the souls of women and children,
Who cry out for a world at peace.

Anguish

I have lived anguish,
For I have passionately felt
Every pang of the breast cancer experience.
I have made it my own.

From the inception of the first malignant cell,
Cancer has infiltrated my womanhood.
Like mold between the walls,
Finally discovered after a long covert residence.

It has been a roller coaster ride,
A ship tossing fearfully in its storm.
Each profound decision terrified me,
Affecting the permanent image of my feminine exterior.

I could not imagine my woman's life without a breast,
Yet I succumbed to the inevitable mastectomy,
Kicking and screaming with rage and violation,
Like a shattered little girl's dream.

I cried for days for my life without beautiful hair,
As I envisioned the ugly prospect
Of seeing myself in the shower and bedroom,
As a freakish amazon billiard ball.

I felt so deeply the loss of external beauty.
My missing breast a phantom shielding my aching heart.
My once silky tresses no longer a royal crown,
Once the outward extension of my motherly soul.

Oh the anguish I have felt!
Painfully robbed of my perceived womanhood!
The nausea, gnawing and ache behind my navel.
The frightened shame of feeling naked to the world.

Yet I have surrendered to each loss as the dreaded night,
Embraced each tear as a channel to an uncertain sunrise.
I have nurtured the anguish so deep in my soul,
That my spirit now radiates with untarnished inner beauty.

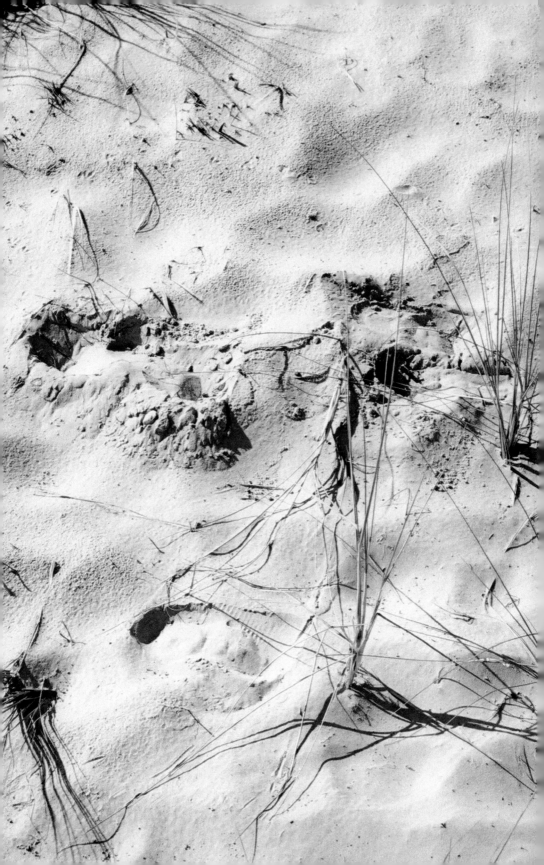

Hair Extension

The essence of my life
Can be compared to my hair.
For the years have been long,
Like the time it takes
To patiently nurture
A beautiful length of silky tresses.

Oh yes, there have been split ends.
Plans have been shunted.
Promises have been broken,
Yet the image has not changed.

Long hair seems timeless.
A passion for natural flow.
Abhorring the rigidity of life's hairspray.
It welcomes ribbons and clips,
And enjoys the delight of creative adornment,
Yet always stays genuine to itself.

And now the effects of chemotherapy
Will springboard an unwelcome transformation.
For I am being forced to discard the old,
Reconnect with the scalp of a baby,
And begin to regrow
New welcomed tresses,
As a fuller extension of myself.

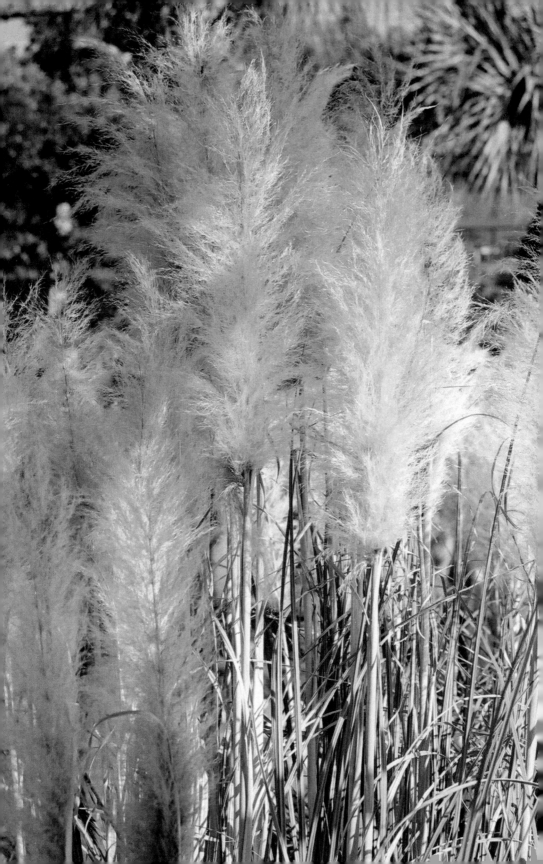

Trans Am

I have breast cancer,

And I also have a Trans Am!

As I tenaciously battle lingering cancer cells

With chemo and radiation,

I slide into the bucket seat

Of my rumbling charismatic carriage,

Press my foot to the pedal of power,

And rejoice in the outward extension of my inner spirit!

For cancer does not have me!

My wig is secure under my Trans Am cap,

As I cruise with open t-tops,

Relishing in the feeling of life as a breeze.

Surrounded by strength and power,

I know the hour will come

When my beautiful hair will resurrect

And once again be blowing freely in the wind.

My soul is like my Trans Am.

It's beautiful and sleek on the outside.

Yet the true essence likes within.

My engine is intelligence and creativity.

The high horsepower under hood,

Will outdistance cancer!

In the "Race for the Cure"

I'm sure….

I'll beat it in my Trans Am!

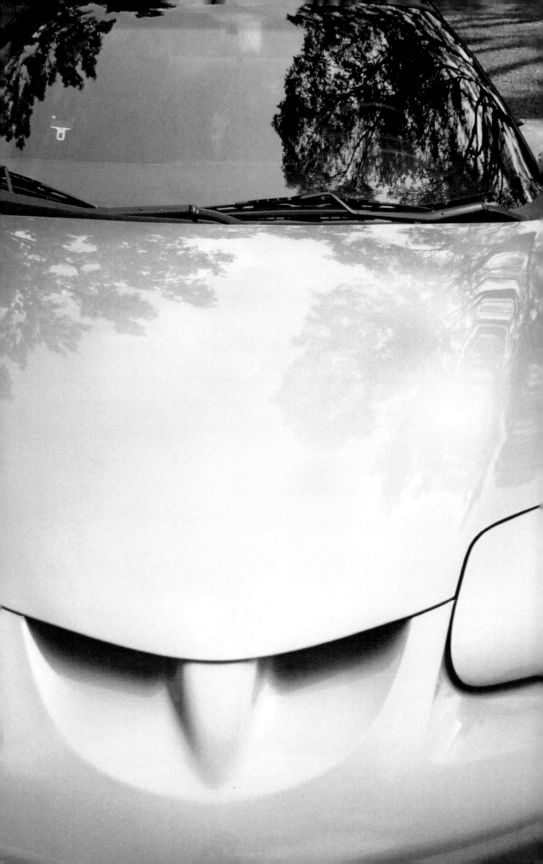

Rear View Mirror

I am sitting silently in my sports car,
Contemplating a beautiful sun-kissed day,
Feeling a breeze glide through the windows,
And focusing my eyes on a green turf cake,
Frosted by a blue puff-filled sky.

I look at the rear view mirror,
And choose not to stare within,
Nor have any need to look back.
I savor the caress in the rich leather seats,
And breathe in the ecstasy of a perfect day.

Tomorrow I will return to this place,
With only one anticipated change.
I will be adorned with a beautiful wig,
To coronate the emotional scars
Of my ongoing journey with cancer.

I will still feel the sun and the breeze.
Still glory in the verdant expanse,
Kissed by God's eternal sky.
I will look at the rear view mirror,
And choose to reject any misguided reflection.

For my life is like this treasured car.
It is meant to move forward,
To rejoice in the power of my spirit,
Without remorse at a discarded past,
That is only a nostalgic glimpse in my…..
Rear View Mirror.

Sampson

Couldn't let a mastectomy cramp my style.
As I struggled to comfort
The frightened little girl of my soul,
I reached out and caressed
A soft little puppy dog
Filled with beans.
I opened his heart-shaped tag
To reveal the name of
Sampson!

Sampson! Sampson!
The biblical hero who lost his hair,
But not his power.
Now I have Sampson
Beside my heart,
Cuddling me within my silky lingerie,
And making me smile
With my clever mammo secret.

Like the Sampson of biblical time,
I have also lost my long silky hair.
My chest now has a queen side,
And a princess side.
My furry bean-filled puppy dog,
My Sampson,
Stays near my heart all day.
He's my clever reminder
That cancer has neither taken my power,
Nor my childlike sense of humor.

Curls... Curls... Curls...

Memories of straight, dark brown hair,
My identity for thirty years.
Silky strands clipped near to the scalp,
On the seventeenth day of chemo.
Short stubs of dark brown hair,
Gradually disconnecting.
Forming a daily wreath 'round the tub drain,
The final balding reality of chemo.

Only a few silky strands
Of dark downy brown
Refusing to succumb,
To the ravaging three months of chemo.
A dark brown "bob"
Of a cute wig with headbands,
My new look for seven months
From the long ago onset of chemo.

A soft silky down of brown,
Begins a thin illusive crown,
Tenuously appearing around six weeks
After the last round of chemo.
I reverently touch the crown of soft down,
Each day breathlessly reveling
In the gradual uncertain resurgence
Of my beloved brown hair.

And in the seventh month,
I triumphantly discard the wig disguise,
And reveal the new phoenix of me in...curls!
Curls, dark brown curls!
God is my hairdresser,
And has given me curls!
To celebrate the spring in my resurrected spirit!

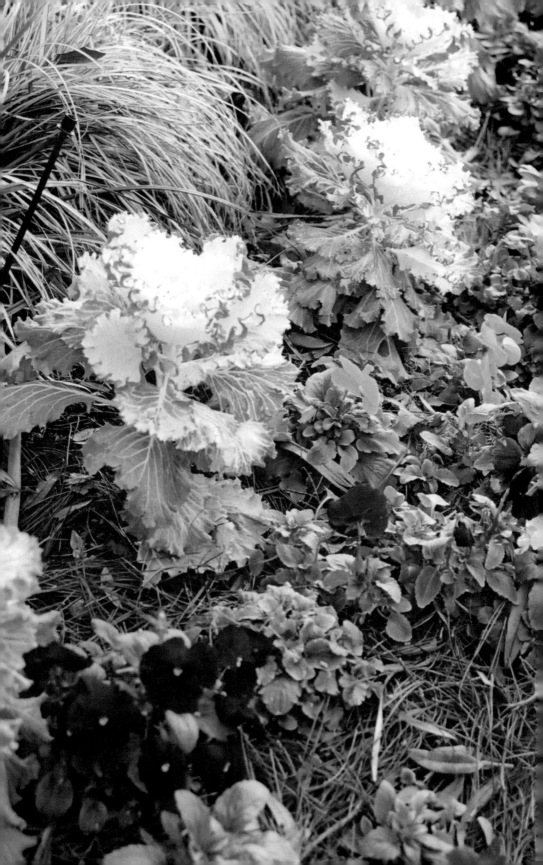

Waiting

I'm waiting on the tarmac.
My plane has left the gate on schedule.
What a charade!
On-time departure!

The airfield is engulfed in fog,
Planes in line along the runway,
Like moist bugs,
Shrouded within a lace curtain.

It's ironic to be here waiting…
Sitting, watching, wondering.
To be belted in, anxious to depart,
Yet patiently trapped…and waiting.

My life of late has been waiting…
Ready to take off,
Yet grounded by my own fog,
In the uncertainty of my flight plan.

Oh, how I yearn for clear skies,
For my intuitive navigation system
To chart my mission and course,
Lifting all fear of the unknown.

Yet part of life's journey is waiting.
Like nine months of a pregnant incubation,
I'm waiting for clearance from the Universe
To ascend into my blue sky of vision.

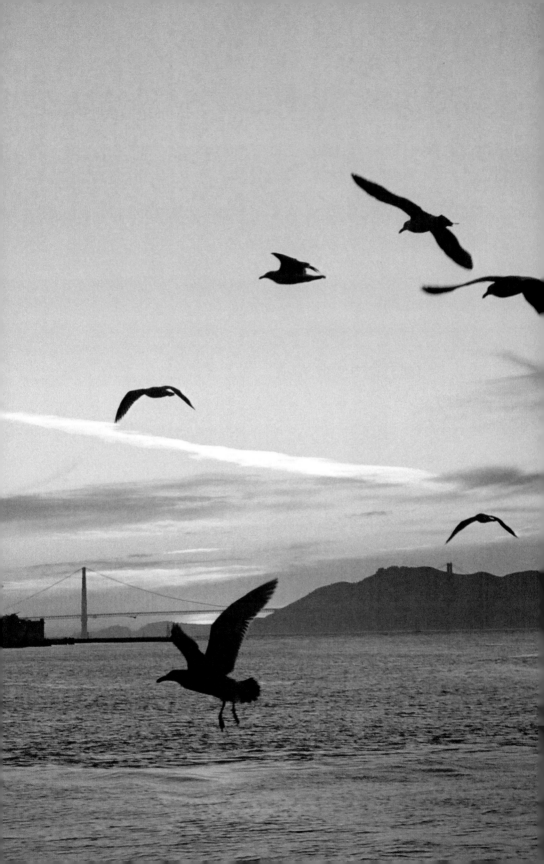

Fog

The edge of night.
The cusp of dawn.
Navigating a lonely highway,
Groping through a tunnel of fog.

I know this road so well,
Bridges that transgress ocean causeways,
Forested borders of scented pine,
Plazas and plantations.

Yet in this new dawn,
All is obscure.
I am thrown into a life of the present
and only one step beyond.

Fog, my life has been in a fog.
The uncertainty of cancer,
Blocks the vision of ahead,
In exchange for cautious creeping in the now.

I've wondered so many hows.
Couldn't envision summer,
Would grieve any good-bye of the cherished,
People and places cloaked in tenuous trust.

Yet with each hour of emerging dawn,
I see farther along the road,
With headlights of confidence on a clearer future,
Beyond the fog of cancer.

Backwards

Have you ever ridden on a train,
With the seat facing backwards?
It is something I generally avoid,
And I didn't know why…until now.

Settled in my forward-facing seat,
I embarked on a significant rail journey.
After a midpoint station stop,
The train pulled out in reverse,
And I was facing backwards.

Backwards, what a limiting position!
Barely seeing out of the corner of my eye
Where I am,
As I focus on the blur of where I've been…
Staring backwards!

It's a reminder of my life of late.
A year of cancer treatment.
Never seeing farther than one step ahead,
Stuck in the now and what I've just passed,
Enduring emotional catch-up.

It's too uncomfortable facing backwards.
For my journey of now is a forward flow,
As I watch cancer's life of uncertainty,
Fade into a blur of profound memories,
'Mid the forward vision of a new tomorrow.

You Came to Me

You came to me
Weary and uncertain,
And I gave you the certainty
In days and rays of sunshine.

You wilted in the heat,
And I gave you the craving for rest,
The chance to listen to your body,
To honor the weary temple of your soul.

You came to me breathless,
And I breathed fresh air into your being,
The crisp, clean atmosphere,
The healing wind of heaven.

You came to my beloved mountain,
Because you sensed I was there.
You entered the cathedral of the Most High.
You came to me, and you were refreshed.

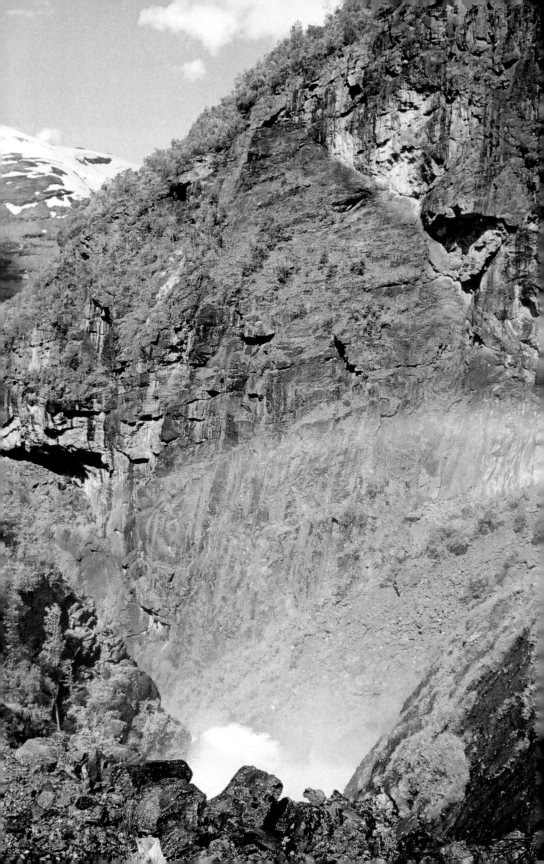

I Understand

Oh, my child,
How I long to hug you,
With the Trinity of my Spirit.
For I know that you need my love,
That you might share it with others.

So, my child,
I send you my love,
In the arms of my emissary,
Who will hold you and listen,
And say for me, "I understand."

For in the everywhere of Being,
I share my caress with so many,
That I appoint ambassadors
To transmit my energy and my Spirit,
So that you might feel my Divine Presence.

The work of the emissary
Is a labor of love,
And when the Spirit is drained and expended,
Be sure that I will send my embrace,
With the voice of one who will say,
"I understand."

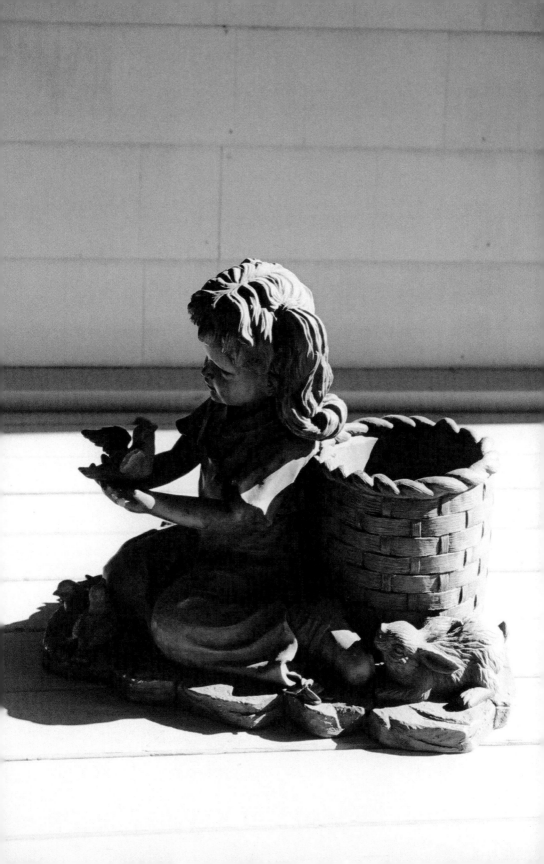

I Have Been Healed

I came to the mountain of majesty,
Burdened with disease's uncertainty.
Yet I breathed deeply the Spirit of God,
And I was healed.

I stepped on the jagged pathway,
Cluttered with granite chips of memory.
They crumbled beneath the strain of my step,
As I firmly connected and was healed.

I breathed the crisp wind of Spirit,
As it flowed deeply into my soul.
I inhaled pure air into toxic cells,
And exhaled the sigh of the healed.

I rejoiced in the throne room of the Most High,
Spinning myself in worship
'Mid such heavenly magnificence.
It surrounded and engulfed my being,
As I honored the blessing of being healed.

I became silent with humility.
Lowered my eyes in dignity,
At the wonder of my divine gift.
For I trust, that….
I have been healed!

MATTERHORN *Reflection*

Kathy Stone continues to return to Zermatt, Switzerland each year to reconnect with the Matterhorn mountain that has been her spiritual inspiration. Since her cancer treatment, she has also written a book of poetry and photographs called *Reflections From the Matterhorn*, which is on sale in English and German in the bookstores of the village of Zermatt. The book is dedicated to Peace and Harmony.

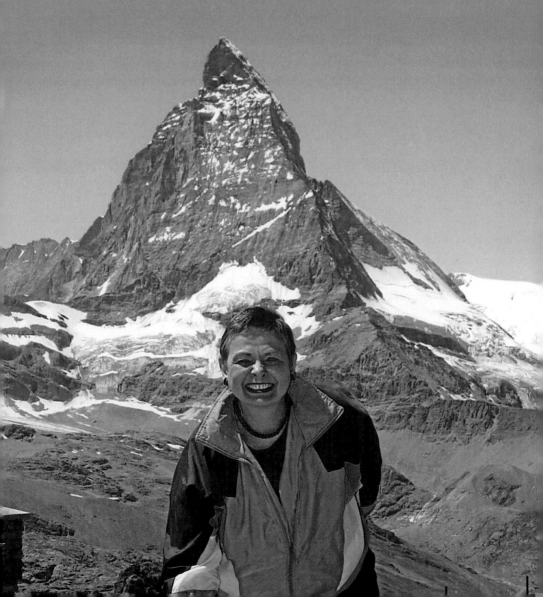

How Sweet It Is!

How sweet it is
To enter the oncologist's office
With a curly head of hair!
How sweet it is
To rejoice at normal blood counts
With each six month follow-up!

How sweet the continued connection
With the oncologist who walked with me,
Through the battlefield of chemo,
To the Christmas holiday onslaught
Of a dangerous white blood cell count.

Let me count the ways my oncologist
Was there for me.
How sweet the sense of confidence 'mid my doubt.
How sweet his patience
for my spreadsheet of questioning.
How sweet the mutual high five
With each semi-annual reunion.

My medical oncologist is a gift,
My living proof of the sweetness of God.
He has touched my soul
to the cellular level,
and celebrates my continuing survival.
How Sweet he is!